The A-List Diet Cookbook

Powerful Recipes That Use Micronutrients To Lose Up To 3 Pounds A Week

By Maximilian Wicks

Table of Contents

INTRODUCTION

Weight gain can occur at any time, it doesn't discriminate, it doesn't care who it takes prisoner. We have seen it time and time again, we try all kinds of diets and nothing seems to work. We are not going to pretend or lie to you and say this is GUARANTEED to work because as with most things, you get back what you put in. Unfortunately, there is no one size fits all. You have to be determined and you have to make the effort. Above all else you have to be honest with yourself. We will give you all the information, the facts, no big scientific words just plain old fashioned English.

We hear you asking "Ok, Yes I want to lose weight, yes I'm determined, why this book? " Because the chances are you have tried most things and it hasn't worked. Maybe you weren't in the right place at that moment in time.

Let us ask you a question, before we do go and get a pen and paper. Don't say you can't find one, if you don't have a pen and paper improvise. It's all about changes and adaptations.

"**Why Now?**" It's a simple question, there is a catch. Be honest, there is no reason to lie to yourself. Remember the saying 'You can run, but you can't hide'. Well, that's never been truer. No one else can see your answer, but you must write it down. The truth! Why now?

On the same piece of paper, write down your weight. It's better if you know your exact weight but if not then an approximate will do. Now take the paper, fold it in half and put it away safe.

You won't be needing that again till the end of the book.

How long will it take to see a result?

Well, that's up to you, some people begin to see results in the space of 3-4 days others after 2 weeks. It all depends on you, your metabolism and your state of mind. All of these we will touch on throughout the book.

Before you take a step further or skim through the book to just pull out highlights (doing that and the chances are it won't work), let us explain exactly what the Micronutrient diet is. That way you can decide if you are willing to commit to this and try your best. Notice we said try your best, be realistic, no one is expecting miracles from you and you won't starve by being on this diet.

What do we hope to achieve in this book?

That's simple! What we hope you will achieve is

Lose weight, increase energy and reverse disease

CHAPTER 1
WHAT ARE MICRONUTRIENTS?

Micronutrients are vitamins and minerals. These vitamins and minerals are vital for the human body. We (humans) don't require these in large amount but we do need small doses of them. They help enable the human body to function properly. They are vital for normal growth, our metabolism and general well-being.

To our knowledge there are 13 vitamins that we know the human body requires along with 10 different minerals, each of them have a specific purpose:

VITAMINS   MINERALS

- Vitamin A
- Provitamin A (Beta-carotene)
- Vitamin B1
- Vitamin B2
- Vitamin B6
- Vitamin B12
- Biotin

- Copper
- Iodine
- Iron
- Manganese
- Selerium
- Zinc

- Vitamin C

- Vitamin D

Macro Elements Required

- Vitamin E

- Folic acid   - Calcium

- Vitamin K   - Magnesium

- Niacin   - Potassium

- Pantothenic acid   - Sodium

Don't start panicking! This won't be an in-depth science lesson. We just want to explain exactly what it is as simply as we possibly can. The list will be broken down as we make our way further into the book.

What you have to remember is that not one single food contains all these vitamins and minerals, therefore they have to form part of a varied diet. That is what the Micronutrient diet is.

What about Vitamin tablets?
We will touch on those in the 'Health Benefit' Section. There are mixed messages about whether they are good or not for you.

There was an expert panel of nutritionist, NGOs and development agencies which identified five micronutrients that were deemed a priority for our health and well-being.
These are the vitamins and minerals which we will mainly be focusing on.

Vitamin A
Folate (Folic Acid)
Iodine
Iron
Zinc
Each of these have not only a specific purpose but are also vital and should be consumed on a daily basis.

What we will do is take each of the Vitamin and Minerals and explain their exact purpose in the human body. Why? Because it will help you understand the exact purpose of micronutrients.

HEALTH BENEFITS

Vitamin A

Experts believe that a lack of vitamin A is a common cause of an unhealthy immune system, not growing properly and blindness.

Over 5 million children across the globe suffer from vitamin A deficiency. That is a large number of children that will go blind and can easily be avoided by a simple change in their diet. Vitamin A is known to for the development of white blood cells.

Folate (Better known as Folic Acid)

Folic acid primarily is found in Vitamin B. It helps increase stability and plays a key role in your metabolism. It also helps aid the production of proteins and the molecules which carry the generic information in your cells. Which in turn help with the formation of your blood cells.

Iodine

We will focus a lot on Iodine as this is the most common deficiency in developed and developing countries. 2 Billion People across the globe have an insufficient Iodine intake. The chances are you could be one of them.

Iodine helps with the production of your hormones and helps maintain a healthy mental state.

Iron

Iron helps carry oxygen from your lungs to your body's tissue. It's the Haemoglobin and is vital to help the enzymes reaction within our body tissue.

If you have Iron deficiency then that basically means that your blood cells aren't functioning properly. This is when people are diagnosed with Anaemia.

It may surprise you to know that along with Iodine deficiency, Iron deficiency is equally as common in both developed and developing countries.

Zinc

Zinc deficiency is part of the immune system. It mainly impacts children in development. Recurrence infections and where diarrhoea is found to be the most common side effect.

MENTAL BENEFITS

By not getting the right amount of vitamins and minerals, you are actually aiding mental health problems. The human body relies on you to keep the nutrients balanced.

Having less energy, feeling anxious and tired all the time. These are all clear signs that your body isn't getting what it needs. You can change that, along with our help we will introduce you to ways which you can alter even just the slightest thing and watch as your body begins to change.

Depression

We don't mean the odd day of the winter blues, we mean serious depression. There are a number of minerals which are closely related to this. You may be on anti-depressants but that doesn't mean you have to stay on them (before coming off any form of medication, please consult your doctor first).

The serotonin and other compounds which are released through the minerals do play a vital role in your mental capacity.

Other mental health disorders associated with deficiencies are;

- Paranoia
- Confusion
- Anxiety
- Fatigue
- Tearfulness

A lot of these can be avoided or reversed if you have them by simply following the micronutrient diet. A careful blend of vitamins and minerals is all the human body needs to stay healthy.

Take all those deficiencies away and you are left with a happy, content, physical body. That in turn will lead to a more positive lifestyle.

> *"Take the first leap in faith*
>
> *You don't have to see the whole stair case*
>
> *Just take the first step"*

Martin Luther King, Jr

Never have those words been truer. You can't see the future, nor can you alter the past but you can live in the now. Change just a simple thing like your diet and tomorrows future will be more positive than the path you are on now. You can't see it right now, we hear you! You've tried everything before this, you feel like you're running out of options. The door isn't closed, let us tell you, the door only closes when you close it. And that applies to a vast range of things in life. Keep Martin Luther King Jr quote in mind and remember it every time you feel you are about to fall. You can do this, it's not as complicated as you may think.

Keep reading and follow the next chapter!

CHAPTER 2
PREPARATION

Chapter 1 focused on exactly what Micronutrients are, that is the main bulk of the science explained for you. Now it's time for the preparation.

The preparation chapter is made up of 3 sub contents

- Possible Side Effects

This highlights some of the main side effects if the vitamin and minerals are not balanced

- The things you can and cannot eat

This is the section that lists the ingredients, I.E – the foods you can by and foods to avoid

- What options are best for you

This is a decision section. Having a pen and paper or somewhere you can record your thoughts and notes would be recommended.

If you wish to recap on chapter one then now would be a good time to do that before you continue reading.

"Start by doing what's necessary; then do what's possible; and suddenly you are doing the impossible"

POSSIBLE SIDE EFFECTS

Contrary to popular beliefs, you can have too much of what's good for you. If the Micronutrients aren't varied they can be dangerous and cause the opposite of what you are trying to achieve.

Health specialist have a recommended intake allowance that they state is enough. What can happen is people take too much and in effect overdose and we want to avoid that. All food and drinks packaging state the nutrition and the % of the daily reference intake.

Don't worry we are not going to tell you to take a close look at every label before you buy it but it is something to be aware of.

Back in 1999, Dr. Furman designed the healthy food pyramid and we are going to use this as a guideline.

Health = Nutrients / Calories (H=N/C)

At least 90% of the daily diet should be comprised of whole plant foods

THE THINGS YOU CAN AND CAN'T EAT

Believe it or not this is the fun part! This is your chance to see if you like what is on the potential menu. Imagine you're out at a restaurant and you see a dish and think yes I want that. What you then have to do is determine whether or not your diet allows you to have it. This isn't as bad as you think and this is a varied diet and alterations can be made. There is that old saying 'a little bit of what you fancy does you good' and that is true but be careful. One sweet unhealthy dessert can reverse what you have already achieved and before you know it you can be back to square one.

Let's begin with what you can eat. No one has a gun to your head and saying you cannot eat this but we don't recommend it and as you have come this far into the preparation you may as well stay a little longer. The only person judging you is yourself. It makes no difference if you tell someone you had a McDonalds or if you keep it a secret. You still had it. This is primarily about choices.

What you can eat under the priority Vitamin and Minerals

Vitamin A

- Carrots
- Spinach
- Broccoli
- Milk
- Egg

- Liver
- Fish

Folate (Folic Acid)

- Egg
- Dairy products
- Asparagus
- Orange juice
- Dark green leafy vegetables
- Beans
- Brown bread

Iodine

- Seaweed
- Fish
- Iodized Salt

Iron

- Lentils
- Red meat
- Poultry
- Fish
- Leaf vegetables
- Chick-peas

Zinc

- Liver
- Eggs
- Nuts
- Cereals
- Seafood

Those are all the things that you can eat. That wasn't as bad as you thought it was going to be, is it? The micronutrient diet isn't about starving yourself. It's all about the balance. You must have a certain intake of one thing off each list every day.

What can't you eat?

Everything else! Mainly processed food. Fast foods are a NO. Though as a treat on a special occasion it won't do you any harm.

Dr. Furman recommends that you consume greens, beans, onions, mushrooms, berries, seeds and tomatoes on a regular basis to maximize immune function and protection against cancer.

We ask that you remember that by doing this diet there is still no guarantee that you won't have cancer or any other disease but it will go a long way in trying to avoid getting life threatening diseases.

WHAT OPTIONS ARE BEST FOR YOU

The best options for you will depend on your likes and dislikes. Did you notice how some minerals overlap in certain foods?

I.E- Eggs – These have traces of Zinc, Folate (Folic Acid) and Vitamin A. By eating one egg you are consuming 2 minerals and 1 vitamin.

You may not like everything on the list but that's the best part, you don't have to. We are all different and there is something for everyone. Simply go through the list and put a tick or an x net to the ingredients. This will help you for your first shop on 'The Micronutrient Diet'.

CHAPTER 3
HEALTH PLAN

You can do eat all the right things and do with near perfection, however, this will not work on its own. There is no magic pill, there are other parts away from the diet that you need to do. This isn't what this book is about? Is that what you're thinking? Then yes in part, you would be right but it would be foolish of us to not include this section. Will all the best intensions and with all the willpower that you possess. This diet won't work wonders solely on changing your diet.

It will help but you won't see the drastic benefits unless you implement this part into it.

What we will be focusing on is primarily your state of mind, once each of these are done on a regular basis and implemented into your daily routine, you will notice some near immediate benefit.

- De stress
- Exercise
- Relax
- Socialize

You need to do these, it is human nature, we were not meant to live in isolation or burden ourselves with endless amounts of stress.

DE STRESS

The most common things are;

- **Work**

Work is definitely up there as one of the highest stress causes. A study by International Stress Management Association found that half the working people in the UK have suffered or are suffering from stress due to work. A quarter have had to have time off work. That is a large number for one small country alone. Stress is the leading cause of sick leave.

- **Relationship Breakdown**

This doesn't necessarily mean with a partner. It could be about anything that you feel you had a relationship with. It could even stem as far back as a link to your childhood. Perhaps an old cuddly bear that has now been lost or destroyed. That relationship has gone and the thought of it not only upsets you but brings stress on. You blame someone perhaps? Maybe it was their fault or not but getting yourself worked up only brings on anxiety, high blood pressure, worry which eventually leaves you feeling stressed, tiered and generally not functioning well.

- **A New Project**

Someone building their dream home is extremely stressful. You have so much to think about day and night and the budget that dreaded budget. However, a new project can be anything from simply a get my act together routine to building skyscrapers. Every new project brings challenges, worry, panic and stress.

- Money

Worried about paying the bills? And debts is also stress related. When you're in debt it's often hard to see a way out and dealing with this is a priority. Whilst your constantly feeling stressed there are ways to help relieve the symptoms but if you are in debt, don't burry yourself in the sand. There are plenty of advice and helplines online. Look them up and go from there.

- **Grief**

Grief is a horrible thing and one hopefully not many people reading this will have experienced on a deep level. It is mostly used for the loss of a loved one but doesn't always limit to just that category. When you lose something you love you grieve for it/them. This is a healing process and not necessarily the one thing that is stressful. However, whilst the grieving process begins other things go unnoticed and a month or two down the line that's when the stress begins. To deal with stress there is no one size fits all but if someone is offering to help then you should take it.

- **Driving**

Anyone who drives at some point or another has found themselves in that stressful moment. You don't know which lane you should be in, you don't know where you're going, someone who has (we hope the person has) got a licence and obviously shouldn't have one or you're late and the traffic seems to be going at a record low speed. You can feel your blood pressure rising and repeat over and over that you won't be doing this again. Yet you probably will do but next time you'll be more prepared.

- Procrastination – Everyone can procrastinate. What is it?

To procrastinate means to put something off, to avoid

something that needs to be done.

That overwhelming feeling you get when you know you have to do something, things like; paperwork, too much cleaning, avoid going to bed because of a late night film. This inevitably leads to something not being done or rushed. The result of that is increased blood pressure, irritable and feeling miserable. That all combined can lead to being stressed.

To avoid this happening, develop a structure. Not just one that looks good on paper but one that is practical. Do a chart, you're not a child your saying? No you are not and no one has said that you are but by doing a chart or a table isn't a bad thing. You can reward yourself for getting something done that may not have gotten done. Researchers reckon that 20% of the human population are chronical procrastinators. This is a fairly high number, if you feel you are falling into that percentage, get yourself out of it. The first step may be to seek profession help. Talk to your doctor!

Being stressed will have a huge impact on your life, whether at work, at home, your social life, even every day things such as doing the laundry can be made into a stressful situation. Getting back In touch with nature is a good way to begin to relieve the highs and lows of every day lives.

Accept the Worst/ Embrace the Good

It's inevitable that things go wrong and an instant reaction isn't always the right one. Ask yourself the following questions:

- What did I learn from it?

- Can I avoid it happening again?

- What good came out of it?

If you can answer them then you can embrace the good. You are living in the Now and acceptance is a key part of now. You cannot alter what happened but you may be able to avoid it happening again. A different perspective is to look at it from a different light.

'I found a way not to do it, next time the right way will happen' Mistakes happen that is part of life but don't self-destruct about it. If you can fix it then fix it and if you can't leave it in the past, taking the lessons learned with you.

EXERCISE

There really is no excuse not to exercise. You can put it off, you can say oh I'll do it later, but really is it that hard to find just 25 minutes a day, every day. I'm sure it isn't. So you have to get up half an hour earlier, is it that hard. That hour you spend drinking your coffee and watching the news. Can't you multitask? We will leave those questions with you, yes you the one reading this book.

Research conducted has proven time and time again as stated by Dr Nick Cavill, a health consultant. That this not only has many health benefits but is a simple and free way to help with stress. Actually if you exercise before breakfast you can burn 20% of your body as opposed to exercising after breakfast. That's what Dr Emma Stevenson and PhD student Javier Gonzalez discovered whilst doing research at the University of Northumbria.

So why exercise? How does that help me de stress?

When you exercise, you feel good. When you feel good, your mind is clearer which, basically means that you will be able to think more clearly. Now this won't make what caused the stress to disappear but will help you think more rationally and that can only be a good thing.

The NHS recommends at least 150 minutes of exercise a week. The benefits are instant. Remember there are so many health benefits (that's not for this book to describe) from exercising.

What sort of exercise do you recommend?

- **A walk**

That simple short 10-minute stroll, now if its spring/summer or autumn going out for a walk can be a lovely thing. Go alone and leave everything behind. If you have children, take them with you. Play I spy with them (that goes for grownups too, it can be a great game).See what you can see, take a camera (preferably not your phone) and take pictures of your surroundings. I bet you'll find things you never knew were even there.

- **Yoga**

Yoga isn't as strenuous as you may think, 15 minutes each day, that's all you need. You can watch and follow classes on YouTube. If you have children, why not ask them to join you? They may not do it right but they may think it's fun and something different to do. You can buy DVDs, watch on line, buy books, and buy an Xbox disk or a PlayStation Yoga disk. There not expensive and if you watch online, there's a high chance that it's free.

?

RELAX

People often underestimate the power that sleeps has. A human body needs to sleep to survive, when you've had a good night sleep you are more alert and less irritable. That is a proven fact.

When you're asleep your mind has time to digest and absorb that day's information. With a lack of sleep you are not performing at your best. The human body on average needs approximately 8 hours of sleep a night. This can be achieved with a healthy sleep pattern. Don't eat anything 2 hours before you go to sleep and your body is still trying to process the food you consumed.

Whichever scenario you fall under, you need to sleep. You will be able to handle the stresses much better in every day life if you can accomplish a good night sleep.

Drink a cup of hot chocolate before you go to bed this will help release the Serotine in your body and relax you. Make sure that your room is dark and not too overcrowded. Sometimes this is unavoidable but if possible make sure it's peaceful and a place to relax.

Another way to relax is to read a book before you go to sleep. Schedule half an hour of reading a novel each night. Not your case files or anything work related.

People often underestimate the power of a hot shower or a soak in the bath.

Bath

A bath should be and feel relaxing. If you have children wait for them to go to sleep that way you can unwind with silence. Put some relaxation music (if you don't like complete silence) on and soak the day away. Light some candles making sure you keep them away from anything flammable. Make sure that the bath isn't too hot. You can also add more hot water once you're in it. Don't let the day ruin your bath. Leave it behind. This is your escapism in a way. Enjoy it!

Shower

The same as a bath accept you're standing up. Well you could choose to sit down but we would recommend you take a shower standing up. Just stand under the hot (not too hot) water and listen to the relaxation music.

The most important thing is to enjoy it, accept that you can't alter the day's events, and if something has gone wrong remember to learn from the mistake made and accept the good that came out of it. If you can't see the good right now, it will appear but at this moment in time, it's time to let it soak away and relax for tomorrow.

SOCIALIZE

The laughter method. This involves simply just laughing, you don't have to go anywhere to do this, and you can be out on your daily errands, at work, at home, at school, pretty much anywhere. Cast your mind back to something that happened that made you laugh so hard, your stomach was hurting and tears were flowing down your face.

You could put a funny clip on YouTube or even watch a comedy show. Get a friend on the phone and just banter.

It is often said that laughter is the best form of medicine, especially when you feel overwhelmed and think you can't handle a certain situation. When you laugh your body releases endorphins which when cooled down allows the body to feel relaxed. It works fast and has lasting effects. When you're in that stress frame of mind, everything can seem too much. Letting it go and laughing you may feel is something you cannot do but you can do it. Even if it only lasts for 20 minutes and for those 20 minutes you are feeling happy. What seemed virtually impossible may suddenly appear to be possible. Sometimes a break and a good laugh is all you need to see things from a new perspective. Focus on the now!

See a show

A lot of the time this will cost you money but it doesn't have to be over the top, we aren't saying go to Broadway or the West End. What we are saying is go and see something light hearted, something that will make you laugh and smile.

You can watch shows online, providing you have a good internet connection that's all you need. The world of YouTube is full of hilarious shows and short clips.

Make a movie night for yourself or with friends. That film you keep saying you're going to watch, make a date with yourself and watch it.

Meet up with Friends / Family

Your always rushing around, that feeling of not enough hours in a day. Make some time to let your friends know that you are still around if they need you. Your family that you don't see very often but were once close to, go and see them or pick up the phone and call. The benefits of a 30-minute conversation with someone you miss and love can help reduce your stress. It's that feeling that someone cares about you. If you're not close to your family or don't have any friends that you would associate with being close friends, turn to social media. Get involved and interact with the world. We are not saying that you should spend 4 or 5 hours a day on Facebook or Twitter but a couple of times a week spending an hour or so certainly won't do you any harm, look at pictures people post and comment, like things and you'll soon find a conversation will begin to follow.

This is another social activity that will depend on your other commitments. If you are working, meet up with your friends for lunch. If this is not possible how about a Skype meeting on your lunch hour. Just because you're not close enough to meet up doesn't mean that you can't interact. With today's modern technology there are many ways to stay in touch and let your family and friends know that you are there for them. Helping someone is a good thing but not to be a people pleaser as this will just add to your stress levels. There is a saying 'A problem shared is a problem halved' If you are worried talk to someone you trust, this can be an instant relief and someone else may see things differently to you.

CHAPTER 4
MICRONUTRIENT 7 DAY MEAL PLAN

Now that you are aided with all the information you need, it's now time to put it in practice. We have designed a carefully nutritious 7 day meal plan. This is a sample plan, you are free to make any modifications as long as it falls under the main priority vitamins and minerals.

What we would recommend, is that as a rule you should eat the following on a daily basis and is also advised by Dr. Furman

- Consume a large green salad every day, and put some raw onion and shredded cruciferous veggies on top.

- Eat at least a 1/2 cup of beans or lentils each day, in a soup, stew, or top of a salad or in another dish.

- Eat at least 3 fresh fruits a day, especially berries, pomegranate, cherries, plums, and oranges.

- Eat at least 1 ounce of raw seeds and nuts daily, utilizing some chia seeds, flax seeds and walnuts.

- Consume a double-sized serving of steamed greens daily, and utilize mushrooms and onions in your dishes.

BREAKFAST

DAY 1

Omelette Muffins
Serves: 2

Ingredients
Coconut oil or paper muffin liners
8 eggs
1/8 cup water
½ BBQ chicken or cooked lean meat cut into small pieces
2 cups diced vegetables (red bell pepper, asparagus, broccoli and onion recommended)
¼ tsp salt
1/8 tsp ground pepper

- Preheat oven to 180 degrees Celsius
- Grease 8 muffin cups with coconut oil or line with paper baking cups.
- Fill any remaining muffin cups with 1 inch of water so they do not scorch while baking.
- Beat the eggs in a medium bowl and add meat, vegetables, salt and ground pepper.
- Pour the mixture into the muffin cups.
- Bake for 18-20 minutes.

DAY 2

Cinnamon Fruit Oatmeal

Frozen blueberries work well in this satisfying breakfast.

Serves: 2

Ingredients

1 cup water

1 teaspoon vanilla extract

1/4 teaspoon ground Ceylon cinnamon

1/2 cup old-fashioned oats

1/2 cup blueberries

2 apples, chopped

2 tablespoons chopped walnuts

1 tablespoon ground flax seeds

1/4 cup raisins

In a saucepan, combine water with the vanilla and cinnamon. Bring to a boil over high heat. Reduce the heat to a simmer and stir in the oats.

When the mixture starts to simmer, add the blueberries. Remove from heat when berries are heated through.

Cover and let stand for 15 minutes until thick and creamy.

Mix in apples, nuts, flax seeds, and raisins.

■■■

DAY 3

Green Smoothie

Start your day with this smooth and creamy concoction.

Serves: 2

<u>**Ingredients**</u>

3 ounces baby spinach or kale

2 ounces romaine lettuce

1 banana

1 cup frozen or fresh blueberries

1/2 cup unsweetened soy, hemp or almond milk

1/2 cup pomegranate juice

1 tablespoon ground flaxseeds

Blend all ingredients in a high-powered blender until smooth and creamy.

■■■

DAY 4

Banana Oat Bars

A healthy treat that's sure to be a crowd pleaser.

Serves: 8

<u>**Ingredients**</u>

2 cups quick-cooking rolled oats (not instant)

1/2 cup unsweetened shredded coconut

1/2 cup raisins or chopped dates

1/4 cup chopped walnuts

2 large ripe bananas, mashed

3/4 cup finely chopped apple

2 tablespoons ground flax seeds

- Preheat oven to 350 degrees F.
- Mix all the ingredients in a large bowl until well combined.
- Press into a 9-by-9-inch baking pan and bake for 30 minutes.
- Cool on a wire rack. When cool, cut into squares or bars.

Note: For Banana Oat Spice Bars, mix in:
1/2 teaspoon ground cinnamon
1/4 teaspoon allspice
1/4 teaspoon ground cloves
1/4 teaspoon ground nutmeg
1/8 teaspoon black pepper

Day 5

Green fritters

A quick, easy and healthy breakfast that will keep you satisfied until lunch, with eggs, broccoli and courgettes.

Serves: 2

Ingredients

140g courgettes, grated

3 medium eggs

85g broccoli florets, finely chopped

Small pack dill, roughly chopped

3 tbsp gluten-free flour or rice flour

2 tbsp sunflower oil, for frying

- Squeeze the courgettes between your hands to remove any excess moisture, or tip onto a clean tea towel and twist it to squeeze out the moisture.
- Beat the eggs in a bowl, add the broccoli, courgettes and most of the dill, and mix together. Add the flour, mix again and season.
- Heat the oil in a non-stick frying pan. Put a large serving spoon of the mixture in the pan, then add 2 more spoonful's so you have 3 fritters. Leave for 3-4 minutes on a medium heat until golden brown on one side and solid enough for you to flip over, then flip over and leave to go golden on the other side. Repeat to make 3 more fritters (there is no need to add any more oil to the pan after the first batch). Scatter with the remaining dill to serve.

DAY 6

Pumpkin Spiced Oatmeal

Ingredients

Serves: 3-4

1 cup   Old fashioned oats, dry

2 cups   1 % milk

1/2 cup Pumpkin puree

2 T   Honey or agave

1/4 t   Cinnamon, ground

1/4 t   Nutmeg, ground

- In a medium size sauce pan, combine oats, milk, pumpkin puree, honey, cinnamon and nutmeg. Stir to combine.
- Cook oats on low heat, stirring continuously for 5-7 minutes until oats are thoroughly cooked and mixture begins to thicken.
- Serve warm and top with some, none, or all of the suggested toppings!

■■■

DAY 7

Super Seed Porridge

Serves: 2

Ingredients

90g (3oz) rolled oats

360ml vanilla soya milk

1 apple, peeled, cored and chopped

190g (7oz) mixed berries

40g (1 ½ oz) raisins

1 tbsp sunflower seeds

1 tbsp ground flax seeds

1 tbsp ground hemp seeds

½ tsp ground cinnamon

Cook oats in a pan using soya milk instead of water. Add remaining ingredients and stir.

LUNCH

DAY 1

Fish Fingers

Aim to at least have two portions of fish per week. This one lunch is 1 portion.

Makes 5 fish fingers
Ingredients
2 pieces of flake (or white fish)
½ cup almond meal
½ cup coconut flour
2 eggs
Olive oil for frying

- Grab three bowls and in one, place the eggs, in another the coconut flour and another the almond meal

- Whisk the eggs and cut the two pieces of fish into five or six strips

- Dip the fish into the egg mixture, then followed by the coconut flour to coat, back to the egg mixture and finally over to the almond meal to crumb.

- Place on a plate and repeat the process for all fish pieces.

- Place two tablespoons of olive or coconut oil into a pan and heat, then slowly add the crumbed fish.

- Cook until golden brown and flip. When the whole fish finger is cooked, place on a plate to cool.

■■

DAY 2

Cabbage Salad

Serves: 4

Ingredients

For the Salad

2 cups green cabbage, grated

1 cup red cabbage, grated

1 cup savoy cabbage, grated

1 carrot, peeled and grated

1 red pepper, thinly sliced

1/4 cup dried currants

2 tablespoons raw pumpkin seeds

2 tablespoons raw sunflower seeds

1 tablespoon unshelled sesame seeds

For the Dressing

1/3 cup unsweetened soy, almond or hemp milk

1 apple, peeled and sliced

1/2 cup raw cashews or 1/4 cup raw butter

1 tablespoon balsamic vinegar

1 tablespoon dried currants

1 tablespoon unshelled sesame seeds, lightly toasted

- Mix all salad ingredients together.
- In a high powered blender, blend non-dairy milk, apple, cashews and vinegar and toss with salad.
- Garnish with currants and lightly toasted sesame seeds.
- Lightly toast sesame seeds in a pan over medium heat for 4 minutes, shaking the pan frequently.

  Note: This is good made a day ahead to allow flavours to marinate.

■■■

DAY 3

Russian Fig Dip

This dressing is great on steamed vegetables, Try it!

Serves: 2

Ingredients

1/3 cup no-salt-added or low sodium pasta sauce

1/3 cup raw almonds

2 tablespoons raw sunflower seeds

3 tablespoons of balsamic vinegar

1 tablespoon raisins or dried currants

Blend all ingredients in a food processor or high-powered blender until smooth.

■■■

DAY 4

Mixed Greens and Strawberry Salad

Spinach and strawberries are great together, different we know but give it a try!

Serves: 3

Ingredients

For the Salad:

1 head (about 6 cups) romaine lettuce

5 ounces (about 5 cups) baby spinach

4 cups sliced strawberries, fresh or frozen, defrosted

For the Dressing:

1/4 cup raw cashews

1/3 cup unsweetened soy, hemp or almond milk

1 apple, peeled and cored

2 tablespoons dried currants or raisins

- Pile the lettuce and spinach leaves on a plate and lay the strawberries on top.
- To make the dressing, blend ingredients in a high-powered blender until smooth.
- Drizzle dressing over the greens and berries.

DAY 5

Quick Moroccan Cauliflower Stir-Fry

You can have a deliciously satisfying stir-fry on the table in minutes. All you need is a carton of Moroccan Chickpea and a few high-nutrient veggies!

Serves: 2

Ingredients

1 medium onion, thinly sliced

1 cup sliced mushrooms

2 cups sliced kale, packed

3 cups (about 1/2 head) chopped cauliflower (chopped into 1 inch pieces)

- Heat 2-3 tablespoons water in a large sauté pan and water sauté onion for 2 minutes.
- Add mushrooms and sauté another minute.
- Add kale and sauté until kale starts to wilt.
- Add cauliflower and Moroccan Chickpea.
- Bring to a simmer, reduce heat, cover and cook until cauliflower is tender, about 15 minutes.
- Stirring occasionally.

DAY 6

Mushroom Spinach and Thai Salad

Serves: 4

Ingredients

1 medium onion, thinly sliced

6 tablespoons freshly squeezed lime juice (from about 3 limes)

2 tablespoons vegetable oil

Kosher salt and freshly ground pepper

1/3 cup soy sauce

3 tablespoons sugar

2 jalapenos (preferably red), minced

2 cups mixed fresh basil, cilantro and mint leaves, chopped

4 Portobello mushrooms, stems removed, caps sliced 1/4-inch thick

2 tablespoons toasted white sesame seeds

1 pound spinach, rinsed, stemmed and roughly chopped

- Rinse the onions under cold water, then drain. Toss the onions with 2 tablespoons lime juice, the oil, 1 teaspoon salt and 1/2 teaspoon pepper in a large bowl. Let stand until softened, 5 minutes.
- In another bowl, whisk together the soy sauce, sugar, jalapenos and the remaining 4 tablespoons lime juice. Stir in the chopped herbs. Add the Portobello's and half the sesame seeds and gently mix until well coated with the marinade. Let stand until softened, about 6 minutes, tossing occasionally to better incorporate the marinade.
- Transfer half the onions to the bowl with the mushrooms. Toss the spinach in the large bowl with the remaining onions. Transfer to a platter, top with the marinated mushrooms, the remaining sesame seeds and pickled onions. Drizzle with the mushroom marinade and serve.

DAY 7

Kale and Avocado Salad with Sweet and Sour Dressing

Serves: 2

Ingredients

1 bunch of Kale, washed, stems discarded

1 very ripe avocado, mashed using a fork

2 tablespoons lemon

2 cloves of garlic, chopped

3 dates, coarsely chopped

1 shallot, minced

1 tablespoon hemp seeds

¼ cup raw almonds, chopped

Pinch of salt

- Place kale and avocado in a bowl. Using your clean hands, knead them for 2 to 3 minutes.
- To make the dressing, whisk lemon, garlic, dates and shallot in a bowl until combined.
- Drizzle kale and avocado combination with the dressing and toss to coat evenly.
- When ready to serve, sprinkle hemp seeds and almonds as desired.

EVENING MEAL

DAY 1

Coconut Prawns
Serves: 5 (six prawns is one serve)

Ingredients

16 prawns (peeled and deveined)
180 ml canned coconut milk
3 eggs, whisked
1/3 cup coconut flour
1 cup unsweetened shredded coconut
3 tablespoons yellow curry powder
1 teaspoon cayenne pepper
½ teaspoon sea salt
½ teaspoon black pepper
1 garlic paste
1 tablespoon macadamia oil
1 lime, juiced

- Whisk eggs in a bowl.
- Mix the coconut flour with two tablespoons of curry powder, salt and pepper in another bowl.
- In a third bowl add just the shredded coconut.
- Lay all three bowls in a line. Firstly, dip a prawn in the egg, coat with the coconut flour, then finish off dipping it in to the shredded coconut.
- Once all the prawns are covered, heat up a large pan and add one tablespoon of curry powder. Mix together and cook for one minute.
- Now add the prawns.

- Cook on book sides for about 2-3 minutes. Serve with a squeeze lime.

■■

DAY 2

Luxury steak burger with artichokes and olives

Serves: 4

Ingredients

600g low fat minced beef (maximum fat 10%, or minced lean sirloin/rump steaks)

1 tablespoon capers (drained and finely chopped)

35g sun-dried tomatoes (well drained, finely chopped)

1 tablespoon olive oil

2 teaspoons crushed black peppercorns

400g tinned artichoke hearts in water (well drained)

2 cloves garlic (peeled and crushed)

2 tablespoons fresh parsley (finely chopped)

Juice of half a lemon

25g black olives (stoned and chopped)

- Put the minced beef or minced steak into a mixing bowl and add the capers and sun-dried tomatoes. (You can season with a little salt just before cooking.) Divide into 4 equal portions and press the burgers in the crushed black peppercorns, coating all sides.

- Cut each artichoke heart into 2 or 4 pieces depending on the size of them. Put the olive oil into a frying pan over a gentle heat and then add the garlic and the artichokes, sauté them for 2 to 3 minutes until the garlic is cooked and the artichokes are heated through; then stir in the lemon juice, parsley and black olives. Remove from the heat, cover and keep warm.

- Heat up a heavy ridged griddle pan or frying pan, spray with some low-fat spray and then pan-fry the burgers until cooked to taste, 2 to 3 minutes on each side for medium rare and longer for medium and well done.

- Serve the burgers on individual plates, and then spoon the artichokes in their dressing over the burgers, and garnish with fresh parsley. If not on a diet, pita breads make a great accompaniment.

- -

DAY 3

Smoky Mexican stir fry with chicken

Serves: 1

Ingredients

Spicy Chipotle Chilli Paste, 15g

Edamame Bean Vegetable Stir Fry, 100g

Fry Light - Sunflower Oil Spray*, 4 spray

Chicken Breast Fillets Skinless & Boneless, 75g

Optional: 150g vegetable stir fry mix (in place of Edamame Bean Vegetable Stir Fry)

- Cut the chicken breast into strips and add the spicy chipotle chilli paste, using your hands mix it in well to make sure all the chicken strips are covered in the paste. Set aside for 1 hour to marinade.

- When you are ready to cook, heat up a wok and then add 2 sprays of oil, add the chicken and fry for 3 to 5 minutes, stirring all the time until the chicken is cooked. Take the chicken out of the pan and set it aside.

- Add 2 more sprays of oil to the wok and add the Edamame Bean Vegetable Stir Fry mix, stirring all the time, cook it over a medium to high heat until it is cooked, but still crunchy, then add the chicken and cook for a further 2 to 3 minutes, stirring all the time. Serve immediately and on non-fast days.

DAY 4

Chinese Garlic, Ginger & Honey Chicken with Noodles

Serves: 1 to 2
Ingredients

1 x 125g chicken breast fillet (boned and skinless, diced)

4 teaspoons sweet chilli stir fry sauce

1 1/2 teaspoons runny honey

3 cloves fresh garlic (peeled and finely diced)

1" (2.7cms) fresh ginger root (peeled and grated)

1 tablespoon water

1 medium spring onion (trimmed and cut into slanted slices)

Medium Egg Noodles (30g precooked rice noodles per portion)

- Preheat the oven to 180C/350F. Select a sturdy oven dish – preferably non-stick.

- Place the diced chicken breast into the baking dish. Mix the honey, sweet chilli stir-fry sauce, water, and grated ginger & crushed garlic together in a measuring jug.

- Pour the honey mixture over the chicken breasts, stirring them around in the cooking sauce. Season with salt and freshly ground black pepper to taste and bake in the oven for 10 to 15 minutes. You can also stir-fry them in a wok instead if baking: Heat up a wok and add the diced chicken breast – dry fry them briefly to give them a bit of colour and then add the cooking sauce, mix well and cook for about 10 minutes over a medium heat.)

- Garnish with the sliced spring onions and serve with egg noodles or steamed fresh vegetables, or stir-fry vegetables.

- 200 calories per portion WITH the egg noodles and only 98 calories without the egg noodles.

DAY 5

Thai Vegetable Curry

A great way to introduce someone to Nutritarianism Cuisine!

Serves: 8

Ingredients

4 cloves garlic, finely chopped

2 tablespoons finely chopped fresh ginger

2 tablespoons chopped fresh mint

2 tablespoons chopped fresh basil

2 tablespoons chopped fresh cilantro

2 cups carrot juice (2 pounds carrots, juiced)

1 red bell pepper, seeded and thinly sliced

1 large eggplant, peeled, if desired & cut into 1 inch cubes

2 cups green beans, cut in 2 inch pieces

3 cups sliced shiitake mushrooms

1 (8 ounce) can bamboo shoots, drained

2 tablespoons no-salt seasoning blend, adjusted to taste

1 teaspoon curry powder

2 cups watercress leaves, divided

3 tablespoons unsalted natural chunky peanut butter

1 pound firm tofu, cut into 1/4 inch thick slices

1/2 cup light coconut milk

1/2 cup chopped raw cashews

Un-chopped mint, basil or cilantro leaves, for garnish (optional)

- Place the garlic, ginger, mint, basil, cilantro, carrot juice, bell pepper, eggplant, green beans, mushrooms, bamboo shoots, curry powder, and 1 cup of the watercress in a wok or large skillet.
- Bring to a boil, cover and simmer, stirring occasionally, until all the vegetables are tender.
- Mix in the peanut butter. Add the tofu, bring to a simmer, and toss until hot.
- Add the coconut milk and heat through.
- Top with the remaining 1 cup watercress and the cashews.
- Garnish with mint, basil or cilantro leaves, if desired.

Note: This can be served over brown rice or quinoa.

DAY 6

Thai Longevity Stew

Serves: 4

Ingredients

6 cloves garlic, chopped

2 tsp minced ginger

1½ tbsp minced jalapeno pepper

3 leeks, chopped

140g (5oz) chopped mushrooms

70g (2 ½ oz) grated cabbage

70g (2 ½ oz) grated carrots

100g (3 ½ oz) sugar snap peas

120g (4 oz) no sugar or salt peanut butter

250ml vegetable stock

120ml soya, hemp or almond milk

40g (1 ½ oz) shredded coconut

Juice of 1 lime

Cayenne pepper to taste

2 tbsp chopped coriander for garnish

- Cook ginger, garlic, jalapeno pepper, leeks and mushrooms in 2 tbsp water over medium heat for 5 minutes.
- Add the carrots, cabbage, sugar snap peas and a little more water and cook until tender.
- In a small bowl, mix peanut butter and some of the vegetable broth to make a smooth sauce. Add to the stew with soya milk, coconut and lime juice.
- Add cayenne pepper to taste and serve hot, sprinkled with coriander.

DAY 7

Harvest Skillet Popped Lentils

Serves: 2-3

Ingredients

1 15oz can lentils, rinsed well in cool water and drained

Fine black pepper - add to taste

Salt to taste (if lentils are unsalted in can)

1/4 cup finely chopped parsley (a few generous pinches per cup of lentils)

1 tsp extra virgin olive oil (or to taste - this helps with the crispy edges while cooking)

Cayenne (optional, add a pinch for extra spicy lentils)

- Open your can of lentils and drain liquid. Rinse the lentils in cool water very well. Then drain all the excess water by tossing the lentils in a large bowl strainer. I use a fine mesh strainer. Fluff the lentils a bit so they are as dry as possible. Pat them dry with a paper towel if needed.
- Warm a large skillet over high heat. Add 1/2 - 1 tsp of extra virgin olive oil. Spread around pan.
- When oil is hot, add about 3/4 cup of lentils. Move them through the oil a bit and let them sit there sizzling in the pan. They will start to plump up and almost look like they are about to pop. Shake the pan a bit to toss the lentils for even cooking.
- After about a minute, shake about 1/8 tsp (or to taste) of fine black pepper over the lentils. You can also add some salt if your canned lentils were not salted (check the can). Toss the lentils with the pepper and continue cooking. You can also add in the optional cayenne if you want extra spicy lentils. (You can even add other varieties of spices! Chipotle powder, garlic powder, turmeric, nutritional yeast, curry powder, onion powder... Anything really.)

- You will know the lentils are ready when they look nutty, toasty and the edges are browned and dried. For the last minute of cooking, add in a few pinches of the chopped parsley and toss in pan to wilt with the lentils. Add more spices if desired too.
- Remove these lentils and repeat the process with the remaining uncooked lentils.

Serve warm or cool in fridge for serving cool and adding to salads, lentil toast and more.

DESSERT

DAY 1

Blueberry upside down cake

One slice per serve
Ingredients
¼ cup coconut oil
2 cups of blueberries
1 cup almond flour
½ cup coconut milk
¼ cup coconut flour
2 tablespoons raw honey
3 eggs
1 tablespoon cinnamon
1 tablespoon vanilla extract or a vanilla bean
½ teaspoon baking powder

- Preheat oven to 200 degrees Celsius
- Pour coconut oil in the cake pan
- Add blueberries in the cake pan, covering the entire base
- Heat cake pan and blueberries in the oven for 5 minutes.
- While the blueberries are warming through, combine the rest of the ingredients in a bowl and mix.
- Next add the cake batter to the pan with the blueberries and spread until even.

- Place the cake tin in the oven and bake for 20 minutes.
- Once cooked, remove cake from the oven and let cool for 10 minutes before flipping the cake from the tin onto a serving tray.

DAY 2

Chocolate Cherry Ice Cream

Cocoa powder and cherries make a winning combination. They taste great together and both are packed with powerful antioxidants. Cherries contain anti-inflammatory anthocyanin and cocoa contains heart-healthy flavones.

Serves: 2

Ingredients

1/2 cup vanilla soy, hemp or almond milk

1 tablespoon natural, non-alkalized cocoa powder

4 regular dates or 2 Medjool dates, pitted

1 1/2 cups frozen dark sweet cherries

Blend all ingredients together in a high-powered blender or food processor until smooth and creamy.

■■

DAY 3

Greens Smoothie

Serves: 2

Ingredients

3 ounces baby spinach or kale

2 ounces romaine lettuce

1 banana

1 cup frozen or fresh blueberries

1/2 cup unsweetened soy, hemp or almond milk

1/2 cup pomegranate juice

1 tablespoon ground flaxseeds

Blend all ingredients in a high-powered blender until smooth and creamy.

■■■

DAY 4

Banana and Berry Fruit Salad

Serves: 8

Ingredients

350g strawberries, hulled and quartered

330g blueberries

100g caster sugar

2 tablespoons lemon juice

4 bananas

Mix the strawberries and blueberries together in a bowl,

sprinkle with sugar and lemon juice and toss lightly. Refrigerate until cold, at least 30 minutes. About 30 minutes before serving, cut the bananas into 1.75cm thick slices and toss with the berries.

Ingredient Note

Red raspberries can be substituted for the strawberries. The lemon juice acts as a preservative so that the bananas don't turn brown.

■■

DAY 5

Pear and Ginger Cake

Serves: 8

Ingredients

30g unsalted butter, melted

4 tablespoons golden syrup

4 tablespoons dark brown soft sugar

1 (415g) tin pear halves, well drained

60g pecan halves

415g ginger cake mix

- Preheat oven to 180 C / Gas 4. Mix the melted butter, golden syrup and dark brown soft sugar in a 23cm round cake tin.
- Slice pear halves in half lengthways. Place a pecan in the centre of each pear quarter. Place pears cut side down in

the cake tin, arranging them like spokes radiating from the centre of the tin. Sprinkle any remaining pecans around the pears.

- Prepare the cake mix according to package directions and pour over the pears and pecans in the cake tin.
- Bake 40 minutes in the preheated oven or until a knife inserted in the centre comes out clean. Cool slightly before turning out onto a serving dish.

■■■

DAY 6

Black Cherry Sorbet

Serves: 3

Ingredients

420g (14 oz) frozen black cherries

250ml vanilla soya, hemp or almond milk

1 frozen ripe banana

50g (1 ½ oz) walnuts

3 pitted Medjool dates

Blend all the ingredients and serve.

■■■

DAY 7

Peach and Cherry Quinoa Crumble

Serves: 6-8

Ingredients

4 peaches, chopped

1¾ cup cherries, halved & <u>pitted</u>

2 tablespoons honey

1 tablespoon + 1 teaspoon coconut oil

1 teaspoon vanilla extract

½ teaspoon almond extract

½ cup red quinoa, rinsed

½ cup almond flour

½ teaspoon cinnamon

- Pre-heat oven to 375 degrees.
- Combine peaches and cherries in a large bowl.
- Whisk together honey, 1 tablespoon of the coconut oil (melt the coconut oil if it's not already liquid), and the extracts in a small bowl and pour over the fruit mixture, tossing to coat it thoroughly.
- Pour the fruit into a baking dish.
- In another small bowl combine the quinoa, almond flour, cinnamon and the remaining teaspoon of coconut oil. With your fingertips, combine the mixture so that it loosely forms crumbs (the coconut oil will help it do this).
- Sprinkle the mixture over the top of the fruit in the baking dish and bake for about 30 minutes until the top is slightly browning/crisping and the fruit is bubbly.
- Remove from oven, let cool for 15-20 minutes before serving.

Serve warm. Ice cream on top is a great idea too!

■■■

Did you notice on day 3, that Green Smoothie is mentioned twice? The reason for that is to show you the flexibility of this diet and as you made enough for 2 in the morning, you can place one in your fridge for a dessert later on after your evening meal. You only need 1 smoothie for breakfast.

CONCLUSION

Our body's (human bodies) need Vitamins and minerals in order to survive. It is our job to feed the nutrients that our body need. These are a few examples of what can happen from vitamin and mineral deficiencies:

- **Scurvy –** Lack of Vitamin c
- **Blindness –** Lack of Vitamin A
- **Rickets –** Lack of Vitamin D

What happens when are bodies get enough micronutrients. Some examples (There are hundreds of examples out there) of these benefits:

- **Strong bones -** calcium, vitamin D, vitamin K, magnesium, and phosphorus
- **Prevents birth defects –** Folate (Folic Acid)
- **Healthy teeth.** The mineral fluoride

We mentioned earlier Vitamin Tablets or substitutes and did we recommend them? We would say no we don't, you should be able to manage your vitamin and mineral intake solely on the food which you eat. However, always consult your doctor or pharmacist first.

Now that you have read all the book and have a good understanding of what it involves. Do you remember where you put that piece of paper which you wrote on whilst reading the introduction? Go and get it and read what you put. Do you still think it's realistic? Yes! That's great news, now fold it back up and put it away. Come back to it in 1 month and see the progress you have made.

BONUS MEAL

Broccoli Mushroom Casserole

Serves: 5

Ingredients

3 cups fresh or frozen broccoli florets

8 ounces mushrooms, cleaned and sliced

1 1/2 cups cooked kidney beans or 1 (15 ounce can) low sodium or no-salt-added kidney beans, drained

3 cups cooked brown rice

- Pre-heat oven to 350 degrees F.
- Thaw frozen broccoli or if using fresh, steam for 10 minutes or until crisp tender.

- Sauté mushrooms until tender and most of the liquid is cooked off.

- Combine all ingredients in a 2 quart casserole.

- Bake for 20 minutes or until heated through.

DID YOU ENJOY THIS BOOK?

I want to thank you for purchasing and reading this book. I really hope you got a lot out of it.

Can I ask a quick favor though?

If you enjoyed this book I would really appreciate it if you could leave me a positive review on Amazon.

I love getting feedback from my customers and reviews on Amazon really do make a difference. I read all my reviews and would really appreciate your thoughts.

Thanks so much.

Maximilian Wicks

p.s. You can click here to go directly to the book on Amazon and leave your review.

Made in the USA
Columbia, SC
08 December 2021

50729169R00039